A Gluten Free Diet

A quick guide to know what to eat and what to avoid helping you live a Gluten free life; Gluten free recipes included

Sarah Sparrow

PUBLISHED BY:
Sarah Sparrow
Copyright © 2012

Disclaimer

The information contained in this book is for general information purposes only. The information is provided by the authors and while we endeavor to keep the information up to date and correct, we make no representations or warranties of any kind, express or implied, about the completeness, accuracy, reliability, suitability or availability with respect to the book or the information, products, services, or related graphics contained in the book for any purpose. Any reliance you place on such information is therefore strictly at your own risk.

Table of Contents

Chapter 1:   What's Wrong with Gluten

What is Gluten?

Gluten is a protein that is in foods processed from wheat and other grains, such as barley and rye. The purpose of gluten is to give elasticity to dough, which allows it to rise and keep its shape.   In fact, some bakers will use extra gluten in recipes that require expansion and volume because gluten aids in trapping air bubbles during the rising stage.   While baking, gluten hardens in the dough, which makes it keep its shape.   Breads like hot dog or sub buns use higher amounts of gluten to give strength to the hinge in the bread.   However, other foods like crackers use less gluten because they do not expand in the way bread does.

Gluten is most commonly found in bread, and is what gives the chewy texture we are used to. Without gluten, bread is dry and tends to fall apart into a pile of crumbs.   Gluten is also able to soak up fluids, which is why pancakes are able to absorb maple syrup.

Gluten's main purpose is volume.   It allows food companies to minimize their costs while increasing the size of a product.   Bread was the size it should have been fifty years ago; but when the food companies discovered they could increase the size of their product using gluten, they didn't hesitate.   So these companies are pumping their breads and other products full of gluten, but at the expense of the public's health.

Can Gluten Be Addictive?

Some people assume their cravings for pastas, bread and sweets is rooted in a lack of will power.

However, it is more likely that you are eating foods that you are allergic or intolerant to. Without symptoms as severe as anaphylactic response, one can still be intolerant of foods and be completely unaware of it. When your body consumes food that it is allergic or intolerant to, it reacts by producing addictive narcotics called opioid endorphins. When you eat these foods, it creates a kind of euphoric feeling, causing you to crave them more because of the positive feelings they create in you.

Gluten is among the most common foods to which people are addicted. Dependency on food can cause a variety of symptoms, including compulsive overeating, anorexia, bulimia, obesity, and even feelings of depression and anxiety.

Why Should You Go Gluten Free?

For anyone with celiac disease or gluten sensitivity, a gluten-free diet is a necessity. But for others, it is simply a healthy alternative. There are a handful of reasons why people choose to follow a gluten-free diet. By cutting out gluten, you cut out nearly all carbohydrates because you aren't eating breads and pastas. This is a great way to lose those extra pounds, maintain a healthy weight, and cure carbohydrate addictions.

Most people are unaware of the ingredients in all the processed foods they eat. But by eliminating gluten, they discover a new awareness of what they are eating, and what ingredients are in each item. These dieters have to read up on the products they are consuming, or restaurants they choose to dine in. Often times, gluten-free dieters tend to cook at home, rather than eat at restaurants. In most cases, this is a healthier option, regardless of your diet.

Following a gluten-free diet allows you to find new alternatives to foods you have always eaten. Most people only bake with wheat ingredients, but there is a multitude of alternatives that could be used. Many health food stores carry a variety of gluten-free cereals, pastas, breads and even cookies and baked goods, which are a great, healthier alternative to the processed foods we are used to.

Moreover, cutting out on gluten forces you to avoid certain unhealthy foods. For example, any food that is fried is off limits because of its breading. Other foods, like desserts high in sugar and fat are removed from the diet as well. When following a gluten-free diet, you are more likely to eat healthier foods, like fruits and vegetables because they are naturally gluten-free.

Beyond this, a gluten-free diet can help with certain health issues. While the research is limited, it has been shown that avoiding gluten can help with Rheumatoid arthritis, memory loss, joint pain, and even exhaustion. Eating gluten-free can help reduce the risk of heart disease, certain cancers, and diabetes. And because you are likely to eat foods that are full of antioxidants, vitamins and minerals, the body is able to ward off virus and germs.

Chapter 2: Wheat Allergy and Celiac Disease Gluten Sensitivity

What Are the General Symptoms of Gluten Sensitivity?

There are over three hundred symptoms associated with gluten sensitivity, and these symptoms vary between different people. Some experience diarrhea and abdominal pain, whereas others have irritability and depression. These differences in symptoms make it hard to diagnose. In fact, 95 percent of people with celiac disease or gluten sensitivity go undiagnosed or misdiagnosed with other conditions.

Some of the most common symptoms of gluten sensitivity include bloating or gas, diarrhea, constipation, fatigue, joint pain, poor weight gain, headaches, depression and irritability. Other common, but less well-known symptoms are itchy skin rash, tingly and numbness, pale mouth sores, infertility and even discolored teeth. Children who have gluten sensitivity, especially those with celiac disease, have delayed growth.

While the symptoms vary widely, the cause is the same. They cannot digest the protein in wheat, rye and barley. So when their body detects gluten in its digestive track, it tries to destroy the intruder by attacking it. However, because of this self-defense attack by your body, the intestines, particularly the small intestines, are damaged.

Inside the small intestines are small, finger-like projections known as villi, which absorb nutrients from food as it travels through the digestive tract. Therefore, when someone who has gluten sensitivity eats gluten, the villi are damaged as your body tries to destroy it. Over time, as the villi continue to be damaged, making them blunted and shorter, which prevent nutrients to be absorbed easily. Some people have damaged their intestines so severely that they are no longer able to absorb any nutrients at all.

What Is Wheat Allergy and Intolerance?

A wheat allergy is one of the most common food

allergies in children. Put simply, it is an allergic

reaction to foods that contain wheat. However, a wheat allergy should not be confused with celiac disease. A wheat allergy creates an allergy-causing

antibody to the proteins that are found in wheat. Those who have celiac disease react to the gluten protein in the wheat, causing the abnormal immune

system reaction in the small intestines. Immune

systems are designed to protect us from foreign bodies and pathogens like bacteria, viruses and substances that are toxic. When an allergic reaction occurs, the immune system mistakes a good or normal substance for a foreign pathogen and begins to attack it. A person who is allergic to wheat produces antibodies to the protein found in wheat, which causes the allergic reaction. So when the body creates an allergy-causing antibody to an allergen, the immune system then becomes sensitive to it and will attack the protein when it is eaten.

The symptoms associated with wheat allergy include breathing difficulties, hives, nausea, bloated stomach, and an inability to focus. The allergic reaction involves immunoglobin antibodies to at least one of several proteins found in wheat: albumin, globulin, gliadin, and glutenin. The majority of allergic reactions to wheat involve the proteins albumin and globulin, and gliadin and glutenin are less common allergies.

What Is Gluten Sensitivity?

A gluten sensitivity is different than both celiac and a wheat allergy. A non-celiac gluten sensitivity is the term given to people who are not able to tolerate gluten and who develop similar symptoms to celiac disease, but do not have the antibodies and the intestinal damage that is found in those who have celiac. Studies show that non-celiac gluten sensitivity is an innate immune response, rather than an adaptive one or allergic reaction.

Symptoms of a non-celiac sensitivity are similar to celiac disease. However, a main difference is that people with a non-celiac sensitivity experience a prevalence of non-gastrointestinal, or extraintestinal, symptoms, like headaches, joint pain, and numbness of the legs, arms or fingers. These symptoms manifest themselves anywhere from a few hours to a few days after ingestion.

The main difference between a gluten sensitivity and celiac disease is that gluten sensitivity is much less severe.   Those who have sensitivity to gluten will not test positively for celiac disease.   They also don't experience the same intestinal damage that people with celiac disease have.   Those who do have minimal intestinal damage can remedy this by following a gluten-free diet.

Who Develops Celiac Disease?

According to the Celiac Disease Foundation, a whopping ninety seven percent of people who have celiac disease are undiagnosed.   In the United States alone, over two million people have celiac disease.   That is equal to 1 in every 133 people.

For many people, it is a genetic illness.   If one of your family members, including parents, siblings and children, you have a five percent chance of developing the disease yourself.   Celiac is also most common in people of European descent, particularly those from Ireland, Scotland and England.   It is significantly less common in people of African and Asian descent. Those with genetic disorders, including Down syndrome and Turner syndrome, a condition affecting the development of girls, are also more likely to have sensitivity to gluten.

Years ago, doctors believed that celiac began in childhood, but it has been proven now that the disease can manifest itself at any age. While it is unclear what causes the disease to start later in life, some factors that   can set it off include pregnancy, infection, surgery and psychological trauma.

Since celiac disease is an autoimmune disease, it is not surprising that people who have celiac are more likely to suffer from other autoimmune diseases. Among the most common of these other diseases are type 1 diabetes, systemic lupus, thyroid disease, rheumatoid arthritis, and autoimmune hepatitis.

Why Do Different People Get Different Symptoms of Gluten Intolerance?

Different people experience different side effects of celiac and gluten intolerance, which is part of what makes it so difficult to diagnose.   Researchers are working to study what the factors are that create differences in symptoms.   The three factors believed to play a role in the development of celiac are the length of time a child was breast fed, the age a person began to eat gluten-containing foods, as well as the amount of gluten one consumes. Studies have shown that the longer a child is breastfed, the later the celiac symptoms will present themselves.

Moreover, symptoms vary depending a person's age and the amount of damage that has happened to the small intestines. Many adults go years without being diagnosed with celiac or gluten sensitivity. Unfortunately, the longer a person waits to be diagnosed, the greater chance they have of developing long-term complications.

How Does Age Affect Celiac Symptoms?

Infant with celiac usually experiences diarrhea, steatorrhea (excess fat in stools), stomach cramps, abdominal distension, muscle wasting, irritability, and slow growth, or failure to grow. However, these symptoms generally don't surface until cereals with gluten are introduced into their diet.

In children with celiac, symptoms include diarrhea, steatorrhea, flatulence, weight loss, and short stature. When caught in time, children can generally achieve accelerated growth in height when starting the gluten-free diet.   However, if it is not treated, the child will remain short into adulthood.   As some children reach adolescence, they can enter spontaneous remission, and not experience the symptoms until adulthood.   Stress or pregnancy later in life can trigger the symptoms to surface again.

Adults experience many of the same symptoms that infants and children do.   However, not all adults will suffer from diarrhea or steatorrhea, but rather experience either minimal or even no abdominal discomfort at all, such as gas, bloating and abdominal distention.   In addition, they may have fewer other signs of malnutrition, like iron deficiency anemia, bone fractures and abnormal bleeding. Many celiac patients are misdiagnosed with irritable bowel syndrome because of the link in gastrointestinal symptoms.

How is Celiac Disease Diagnosed?

Often times, people with celiac disease are often misdiagnosed with other conditions that have similar symptoms, like irritable bowel syndrome (IBS) or food intolerance. In many cases, celiac is not even considered until after the initial diagnosis has been proven inaccurate by ineffective treatments.

A proper celiac diagnosis studies your medical history, includes a physical examination and lab tests. Blood tests are administered to test for gluten antibodies EMA (anti-endomysial), TTG (anti-tissue transglutaminase) and DGP (Deamidated Gliadin Peptide).

1. Health History

In the initial examination, doctors seek to understand a person's health history. At this time, the following should be discussed:

- Physical and emotional symptoms
- How long symptoms have been present, and if there is a pattern?
- Are these symptoms consistent throughout the day?
- When and how long do you have symptoms?
- Are there other family members with autoimmune diseases?
- Particularly in children, is their physical and emotional health in a normal range

2. Physical Examination

There is also a physical examination. Based on the symptoms a patient is experiencing, the doctor will perform various tests to check for the following:

- Emaciation

- Pallor

- Hypotension

- Edema

- Dermatitis herpetiformis

- Easy bruising

- Changes in bone or skin and mucosa membrane because of vitamin deficiencies

- Protruding or distended abdomen

- Loss of various sensations in hands and feet, including vibration, position and light touch

- Decreased deep tendon reflexes, muscle spasms, bone tenderness and pain—all of which are signs of severe vitamin and mineral deficiencies

- Migraine headaches

- Peripheral neuropathy

There is not a set of standard tests performed to diagnose celiac disease. A number of tests help the physician to come to a conclusion. Here are some of the medically termed serology tests:

- EMA (Immunoglobulin A, anti-endomysium antibodies)
- AGA (IgA anti-gliadin antibodies)
- DGP (Deamidated gliadin peptide antibody)
- tTGA (IgA anti-tissue transglutaminase)

3. Gene Testing

Celiac disease is largely connected to heredity, which means you can develop celiac if you have the genes that predispose you to the disease. Because of this, doctors are now performing gene tests to diagnose the condition. But not everyone who has the celiac disease genes will actually develop celiac disease. Actually, even though 40 percent of the United States population has the celiac disease gene, only about 1 percent will develop celiac. So carrying the gene does not necessarily mean you have celiac.   In fact, the odds are against it!

The process of gene testing is highly complicated. The genes that predispose people to celiac are found on the human leukocyte antigen (HLA) class II complex of human DNA.   These are known as the DQ genes.

Every person has two copies of a DQ gene—one from each parent.   While there are many types of DQ genes, the two most common in celiac disease are HLA-DQ2 and HLA-DQ8.   A recent study showed that 96 percent of people who were diagnosed with celiac disease from a biopsy carry HLA-DQ2, HLA-DQ8, or a combination of the two. HLA-DQ2 is the most common among patients, and particularly in those with a European heritage. Notably, roughly 30 percent of people with

European ancestors carry HLA-DQ2. HLA-DQ8 is considered rarer, and appears only in about 10 percent of the overall population. However, this gene is more commonly found in those from Central and South America.

On the other hand, those with gluten sensitivity, celiac disease genes aren't a major factor. Recent research has found that only about half, 56 percent, of people with gluten sensitivity carry the DQ2 or DQ8 gene. This suggests that these genes are far less involved in developing gluten sensitivity than developing celiac disease. At the same time, these genes showed up more often in those with gluten sensitivity than in the general population; so it can be assumed that they do play a role, but it is still unknown.

The actual gene testing is non-invasive.   A laboratory takes a blood sample, swabs cells from the inside of your cheek, or collects your saliva with a syringe.   These samples are then analyzed by the laboratory, and all provide equally accurate results. However, a positive genetic test does not automatically equal a diagnosis because not everyone carrying the celiac gene will develop celiac.   A positive result will simply tell you that you are at high risk for celiac.

In May of 2011, during Digestive Disease Week, Bob Anderson, MD, and his group of collaborating researches presented results from the first population study that supports the use of a mixture of HLA-DQ gene and blood testing that determines if Celiac disease is present.   This combination of tests could eventually do away with the typical guidelines of a biopsy.   Moreover, the cost of reaching a diagnosis can be reduced by half. This process, which is preferred because of its non-invasive nature, is cost-effective and much more efficient method for diagnosis.

Gene testing can prove particularly useful for family members of someone who has been diagnosed with celiac, as well as young children who do not have a fully matured immune system.

4. Biopsy

A biopsy of the small intestine is performed when clinical signs and positive laboratory testing indicate a probability for malabsorption. This is performed by a specialist called a gastroenterologist. During a biopsy, a small and flexible biopsy instrument is passed through a tube down the throat and through the stomach, and into the top of the small intestine where there are multiple patches of tissue. The doctor removes the tube and examines the tissue samples under a microscope for signs of damage to the small intestine.

Tissue in a normal small intestine looks much different than the tissue in a small intestine of someone who is an undiagnosed celiac patient.   In a person with celiac, the villi, the small, finger-like projections, are almost completely flattened. Moreover, the enzymes found on the brush border are significantly less as well.   Lactase is an enzyme responsible for breaking down milk sugar to be absorbed, and is one of the brush border enzymes. Because of the decrease in lactase, some celiac patients also can't handle milk products, and develop temporary, sometimes permanent, lactose intolerance.

5. Diet

One of the most important steps in diagnosing celiac disease is noting how your body responds to a gluten-free diet. Once gluten is removed from your diet, the majority of the damage to the small intestine is repaired. And it only takes three to six days to see improvement in the intestinal lining, the mucosa. After three to six months, most symptoms disappear due to the mucosa returns to its normal state.

What If You Don't Respond to a Gluten-Free Diet?

It is possible that even after implementing a gluten-free diet, you will still experience symptoms. This is due to several possible reasons. If you are not strictly following the gluten-free diet, and still ingesting small amounts of gluten, the smallest amount can still cause a reaction. You may also have a co-existing condition that causes similar symptoms, like irritable bowel syndrome, bacterial overgrowth in the small bowel and microscopic colitis. Or you may have refractory disease, or complications from celiac. Talk to your doctor if you are still experiencing these symptoms weeks after starting your gluten-free diet.

Chapter 3: The Gluten Free Diet

What Is a Gluten-Free Diet?

A gluten-free diet is simply that—a diet free of the gluten protein. Following a gluten-free diet can be both frustrating and emotionally challenging, but is the only option for those who suffer from a celiac and other gluten-related illnesses.

Is a Gluten-Free Diet Healthy for Everyone?

Without question, a gluten-free diet is necessary for those with celiac.   But others without the disease are growing increasingly interested in the diet as well. In fact, the gluten-free food industry grew 28 percent from 2004 to 2008 alone, according to Packaged Facts, a market research group.   While many of that percent must follow the gluten-free diet, many of them choose this because they believe it to be healthier.

However, this may not be the case.   There is no medical research to prove that the gluten-free diet is actually healthier. On the contrary, going gluten-free when it is not medically necessary could rob your body of essential nutrients like vitamin B and iron, commonly added to the fortified gluten in wheat.

Cutting out gluten certainly can lead to weight loss, but not for the reasons most people claim. Not eating gluten drastically reduces the amount of refined carbohydrates you consume, which is where much of the weight gain comes from. By going gluten-free you are cutting out pizza, beer, burgers, pastas, and other high carbohydrate food choices. Moreover, you are more likely to eat other whole grains and gluten-free flours. To replace the flour-based foods, people choose buckwheat, quinoa, teff and wild rice.

What to Keep In Mind When Considering to Go Gluten-Free?

Before you decide to go gluten-free, don't do it blindly. If you suspect that you have celiac, or another form of gluten sensitivity, you should get a blood test. Then you can discuss with a doctor the benefits and sacrifices of gluten-free dieting.

Don't simply assume a gluten-free diet is healthier. Cutting out gluten will make your grocery bill spike because the gluten-free alternatives tend to cost more. Gluten-free food has not been scientifically proven to be healthier, so you may be wasting your money. Most people eat more fruits and vegetables after eliminating gluten from their diet, which may account for them feeling better, rather than the lack of gluten.

Be careful of the gluten-free labels that you do see. Currently, the Food and Drug Administration does not regulate guidelines for "gluten-free," and some companies use small amounts of gluten in their gluten-free labeled products. Always read the ingredient list and check for wheat, barley and rye, or products made with those plants.

What Are the Nutritional Benefits of a Gluten-Free Diet?

Many foods that contain gluten are heavily processed. These foods, obviously, are not good for you because of all the chemicals and artificial flavors. On a gluten-free diet, you are more likely to eat fruits, vegetables, and other fresh foods. The diet also eliminates a large amount of unhealthy oils and carbohydrates in breads and other pastries. By cutting out gluten, you can reduce your risk for heart disease, certain cancers and health risks like diabetes. Moreover, it can help your body fight off germs and viruses because the foods you are eating will likely have more antioxidants, essential vitamins and minerals. But it is also important to still have a healthy amount of gluten-free starches, like rice, potatoes and gluten-free pastas.

What Are the Side Effects of a Gluten-Free Diet?

After cutting gluten out of the diet, it is not uncommon for those with celiac to begin gaining weight. Many patients are particularly thin before their diagnosis because the damage to the small intestine prevents their body from absorbing the nutrients in food. Once the gluten is eliminated and the intestines repair themselves, the nutrients are absorbed better again. Even if you don't increase the amount of calories you consume, you will likely gain weight. Studies have even shown a higher likelihood for obesity in gluten-free dieters. On the other hand, some people end up losing weight because the diet change may decrease the amount of calories they consume. Exercise and watching your calorie intake will help you manage weight gain or loss you may experience.

Many celiac patients have nutritional deficiencies. To make matters worse, many gluten-free foods are low in vitamin B, calcium, vitamin D, iron, zinc, magnesium and fiber. A study in Sweden showed that adult celiac patients who had cut out gluten for ten years found several vitamin deficiencies in them, as well as high levels of homocysteine, which is a risk factor for heart attacks, vascular disease and strokes. Talk with your doctor about vitamin needs at your annual check-up.

Other side effects to a gluten-free diet include constipation, flatulence and diarrhea. Eliminating gluten and replacing it largely with rice, you also eliminate fiber in your diet, often causing constipation. However, replacing breads and pastas with foods like Quinoa too quickly can lead to diarrhea.

Many people can't digest lactose when they are first diagnosed with celiac. This is due to the intestinal damage from the celiac disease. So when your intestines begin healing, you will once again be able to handle the lactose. Lactose intolerance symptoms include diarrhea, constipation, gas and bloating. So if you experience these symptoms shortly after starting your gluten-free diet cut them out again and wait a few weeks before attempting to reintroduce them. Also try lactose-free or lactose-reduced milk to see how your body reacts to those products. If you don't eat dairy products, be sure to consume enough calcium in other ways.

When you eat gluten regularly, your body probably didn't react to each individual time it was consumed. However, once it is removed, your body will likely have an intense, severe reaction to it when reintroduced. Often times these symptoms are rapid, within thirty minutes; or they may not appear until as late as the next day or two. These symptoms can include diarrhea, constipation, severe abdominal pain, reflux, gas, and even vomiting. Depending on the person and amount consumed, patients could end up hospitalized from the pain, bloating and dehydration. You can also experience joint pain, fatigue, brain fog and feelings of depression because of the gluten.

A lack of fiber is a common gluten-free diet side effect. To combat this, many gluten-free bread companies are producing breads that have more whole grains. Many people suffer from constipation because they are fiber deficient. Try adding alternative fibers to your diet, like whole grain gluten-free bread, beans, legumes, and fresh fruits and vegetables.   Nuts and seeds make great high-fiber carry-along snacks.   Take note that you not add significant amounts of fiber into your diet all at once.   This could upset your digestive tract and cause your stomach to bloat.   If constipation becomes severe or uncomfortable, talk to your doctor about treatment options.

Chapter 4:   What to Eat and Drink and What to Avoid

What Are Gluten-Containing Foods and Ingredients to Avoid?

Following a gluten-free diet can be much harder than people realize.   Gluten is hidden in many foods and products without us ever knowing. Here is a list of foods to avoid while following a gluten-free diet:

- Wheat and wheat-related products. Avoid hydrolyzed wheat protein, wheat starch, wheat germ, etc. Also watch for other names for wheat, like flour, spelt, semolina, durum/duram, graham, couscous, matzah, cake flour and so on. The following items typically have wheat in them, unless otherwise noted as gluten-free:

  - ❖ Bread
  - ❖ Beer
  - ❖ Crackers
  - ❖ Cornbread
  - ❖ Licorice
  - ❖ Many breakfast cereals
  - ❖ Soy sauce
  - ❖ Gravy
  - ❖ Pasta
  - ❖ Pretzels
  - ❖ Pizza

- ❖ Stuffing
- ❖ Fried foods

- Wheat starch is wheat that has had the gluten extracted; but it is possible that traces of it will still be present.   In some countries, Codex Alimentarius, a wheat starch, is accepted on a gluten-free diet; but it is not accepted as such in North America.

- Barley and barley products.   Be cautious of malt flavoring, as the majority comes from barley.

- Triticale, a cross between wheat and rye.

- Rye, which isn't typically hid in any ingredients.

Gluten-Free Ingredient Substitutes and Food

Most foods have a gluten-free alternative, or can be made using gluten-free substitutes. If a recipe calls for flour, you can use wheat-free flour, like cornstarch or other kinds of gluten-free flour. New flours are available, like bean, sorghum and amaranth. Many people miss breaded foods once they start their gluten-free diet. A great way to still enjoy those types of foods is using gluten-free bread or muffin mixes in place of regular bread or cracker crumbs. You can also use potato chips, corn flour or seasoned cornmeal for making breaded foods.

Some foods need thickeners and binders. Most people don't realize how often flour is used in foods like soup to add thickness. Instead, use cornstarch, tapioca starch or arrowroot flour. Or, for sweet recipes, try dry pudding mixes. Salad eaters will be happy to know there is a substitute for croutons; and they're easy to make on your own. Simply take your gluten-free bread, cut them into cubes and then season and fry them as you like. Some people suggest waiting for the bread to get slightly stale (not moldy) before making the croutons; and since gluten-free bread doesn't last very long, this is a great way to use the bread once it reaches the end of its shelf life.

What Alcoholic Beverages Are Gluten-Free?

Most people are surprised to learn how many alcoholic beverages contain gluten. It is often a hidden ingredient that you don't think about when drinking. This is because many types of alcohol are distilled with wheat. The following is a list of alcohols that are gluten-free. However, the list is always changing, so be sure to verify it yourself by checking the ingredients or contacting the manufacturer.

Rum, gin, whiskey, tequila, most wine, and certain vodkas (made from potatoes or corn) are a few of the most common types of gluten-free alcoholic beverages.   However, some flavored alcohols may not be gluten-free, so use caution.

Vodkas

- Smirnoff (non-flavored)
- Absolut Vodka
- Zodiac
- Cold River

Tequila

- Jose Cuervo
- Sauza

- Centinela

Rum

- Captain Morgan Spiced Rum
- Bacardi
- Malibu

Whiskey

- Scotch Whiskey
- Chivas
- Jack Daniels

Wine and Champagne

- Kendall Jackson
- Berringer
- Rodney Strong
- Five Oaks

Beer

- Redbridge

- Bard's Tale
- New Grist
- Rampo Valley Honey Beer
- New Planet Tread Lightly Ale

Gluten-free beer uses two grain plant substitutes: sorghum and buckwheat. Sorghum is a type of grass whose seeds can be harvested as a grain in order to make beer. Buckwheat is not a grass, and is completely different from other grains. Seeds from this annual plant can be used to make flour, and the plant itself can be malted to make gluten-free beer.

How to Read the Labeling of Food and Food Ingredients

Currently, the FDA does not require manufacturers to specifically include gluten on food labels. Because of this, it can be both daunting and dangerous to look for gluten free foods at the store. Some foods are obvious, like foods that contain wheat, barley and rye. However, some foods only contain gluten some of the time. Some labels use the Latin terms for wheat, barley and rye. Keep an eye out for these ingredients, which always mean there is gluten:

- Triticum vulgare (wheat)
- Triticale (a cross between wheat and rye)
- Hordeum vulgare (barley)
- Secale cereal (rye)
- Triticum spelta

The following lists are ingredients that always contain gluten:

- Wheat protein
- Wheat starch
- Wheat flour

- Bulgur

- Malt

- Couscous

- Farina

- Pastas (unless otherwise indicated)

- Seitan

Gluten-free foods can still be cross-contaminated when they come into contact with gluten-containing foods. Often times, this cross-contamination happens during the manufacturing process. This can happen if the same equipment is used to make multiple products. But it can also happen at home if you use utensils or share surfaces between gluten and non-gluten containing foods. If not all people in your household follow a gluten-free diet, you should have two separate toasters for bread. If you have a reaction to something you have eaten that should not have gluten in it, you are probably having a reaction due to cross-contamination.

A Comprehensive Gluten-Free Food List

- Alfalfa
- Algae
- Almonds
- Apple cider vinegar
- Arabic gum
- Arrowroot
- Artichokes
- Artificial butter flavoring
- Baking soda
- Balsamic vinegar
- Beeswax
- Beans
- Blue cheese
- Brown sugar
- Buckwheat
- Butter
- Cane sugar

- Cane vinegar
- Canola oil
- Castor oil
- Champagne vinegar
- Cheese
- Chestnuts
- Chickpeas
- Chocolate liquor
- Cocoa
- Cocoa butter
- Coconut
- Coconut vinegar
- Corn
- Corn masa flour
- Cornmeal
- Corn flour
- Corn starch
- Corn sugar
- Corn syrup
- Corn sweetener
- Cotton seed

- Cotton seed oil
- Cream of tartar
- Curds
- Dates
- Dutch processed vinegar
- Eggs
- Fish
- Flaked rice
- Flax
- Fruit
- Garbanzo beans
- Gelatin
- Glucose
- Grits
- Hominy
- Honey
- Hops
- Horseradish
- Kasha
- Lactase
- Lactose

- Lemon grass
- Lentils
- Maize
- Masa
- Meat
- Milk
- Millet
- Mustard flour
- Nuts (except wheat, rye and barley)
- Oats
- Paprika
- Peas
- Peanuts
- Peppers
- Polenta
- Potatoes
- Potato flour
- Quinoa
- Rice
- Rice flour
- Rosematta

- Saffron
- Salt
- Seaweed
- Sherry vinegar
- Sorghum
- Soy
- Soybeans
- Tapioca
- Tapioca flour
- Taro
- Tarrow root
- Tea
- Teff
- Teff flour
- Tofu
- Vinegar
- Vanilla extract
- Whey
- White vinegar
- Wine
- Wild rice

- Xanthan gum
- Yeast
- Yogurt

Chapter 5:   Cooking and Dining Gluten-Free

The High Cost of Gluten-Free Foods

Anyone following a gluten-free diet knows the cost is considerably higher than a traditional diet.   But they may not realize just how much more they are actually spending.   A recent study in Nova Scotia of fifty-six gluten-free foods found that the average cost of a gluten-containing product was about $.61; its gluten-free counterpart was averaged at $1.71. This means that gluten-free foods, on average, are 242 percent more expensive.

A good way to avoid the high cost is to avoid gluten-free snack and junk foods.   Most of these products, like cookies and crackers, are mostly made with highly refined cheap starches. What's more, they are filled with large amounts of carbohydrates and sugars.

Once diagnosed with celiac, it is important to meet with a dietary consultant. A specialist can help you create a diet based around fruits, vegetables, rice and potatoes. This curbs the need to purchase the expensive gluten-free versions of bread, crusts, crackers and pizza.

You should also make a habit out of reading labels on products. In some cases, there are alternatives to specialty products that aren't specifically labeled gluten-free. Soy sauce is an example of this. While some soy sauce uses wheat as a filler; but others are gluten-free and cost less than those specifically marked as such. These are products you really have to search for.

If you itemize your tax return and your medical expenses for the year total 7.5 percent of your income, you can write off some celiac-related expenses. This way you can deduct the difference of a gluten-free product over a gluten-containing product. Note that you will likely need a doctor's letter to confirm you are a celiac patient, and your need for gluten-free dieting. Make sure you save your receipts in the case of an audit.

A Gluten-Free Kitchen

Cooking for yourself when you follow a gluten-free diet is generally the easiest, safest route to take. There are a few items you should always keep in your pantry. There are many gluten-free flour alternatives, and you should always have some in your house. You should also stock up on various gluten-free baking mixes. Try the different mixes to see which blends you like best. Once you know, you can start making your own, and save money on buying ingredients you already know you don't like!

While your diet will change drastically in what you are able to eat, there are still great snack foods available to munch on. Popcorn makes a great mid-day or evening snack, and is naturally gluten-free. You will have to cut out flour-based cakes and pastries for dessert, but you can still enjoy gelatin desserts, rice crispy treats, and ice cream. There are also plenty of gluten-free alternatives.

Every gluten-free kitchen should have at least one gluten-free cookbook. A good gluten-free cookbook will have good glossaries and descriptions of the gluten-free ingredients.   Some will even provide contact information for celiac support groups broken down by state.

How to Bake Gluten-Free Bread

When baking gluten-free bread, it is important to remember that all ingredients should be at room temperature before starting.   Cold or chilled ingredients will stunt the bread from rising.   For consistent results, it is recommended that you do not make substitutions in the recipe; you should also weigh the dry ingredients on a kitchen scale.

Dry Ingredients:

- 1 cup (4.8 ounces) white rice flour
- 1 cup (3.5 ounces) tapioca starch
- ½ cup (2.6 ounces) sweet sorghum flour
- ½ cup (2.5 ounces) brown rice flour

- 2 tbsp (20 grams) dry active yeast

- 2 tbsp (25 grams) cane sugar

- 1 ½ tsp. (11 grams) salt

- 1 tsp. (3 grams) guar gum

- ¾ tsp. (2 grams) xanthan gum

- ¼ tsp. (1.25 grams) ground ginger

- Optional: 1 tbsp. (7 grams) apple fiber

Liquid Ingredients:

- 3 large egg whites, room temperature

- 2 tbsp (25 grams) light olive oil

- 1 tsp. (5 grams) apple cider vinegar

- 1 cup+3 tbs+1 tsp. (9.66 ounces) lukewarm water

Place the room temperature egg whites in a mixing bowl. For best results, use a stand mixer with a paddle attachment, and beat the egg whites on high for about one minute, or until it is light and airy.

Combine the apple cider vinegar and olive oil on medium speed to the egg whites. Slowly add the rest of the dry ingredients to the egg mixture. Turn the mixer to a low speed and gradually pour in the warm water. Keep beating on low until you have a thick batter. Scrape all the excess batter off the sides of the bowl and mix on high for three minutes.

You will then have a thick batter that will stick to the mixing paddle without dripping off. However, this will not form a dough ball like regular wheat flour dough. Use a spreader spatula to spread the batter in a greased 8 x 4 inch loaf pan; use heavy-duty metal if you have it. To prevent the spatula from sticking, dip it in water several times as you spread it in the pan. Once the batter is in the pan, be sure to get rid of any air bubbles and pockets in the dough.

Loosely cover the batter with plastic wrap and set the pan in a warm, draft-free place to rise for 30-45 minutes.   The loaf should rise to the top edge of the pan.   Preheat your oven to 375 degrees. Place your loaf in the oven for 30 minutes, or until the top is golden brown.   Tent the bread loosely with aluminum foil, and bake again for another 30 minutes.   The best way to determine if the bread is fully cooked is to use an instant-read thermometer. When the internal temperature of the bread reaches 208 degrees in the middle, the bread is finished. Use a spatula or knife to remove the bread from the pan immediately after taking it out of the oven. Cool the bread on a wire rack until completely cooled.

Chapter 6:   Traveling and Eating Out

The Challenge of Traveling on a Gluten-Free Diet

Traveling can be stressful for anyone.   But those with celiac and gluten intolerance face an even bigger challenge.   When the rest of your travel companions can stop at any fast food chain or airport food vendors, you find yourself looking at menu on top of menu full of burgers, pastas and fried foods.   But there are a few tips and tricks to keep yourself from starving as you travel.

Most airlines have done away with food service on flights.   Since then, on most flights you are now allowed to bring food along with your carry on. Currently, with the restrictions on liquids, only solid foods are allowed on board.   Try bringing some

fresh fruits or vegetables in a grocery bag.
Bringing a note from your doctor about your diet
needs is also a good idea. You can take cold items,
like hard boiled eggs and lunch meats in hot/cold
to-go bags that you can get at most grocery and
whole food stores. Also cut up fruits and
vegetables into bite-size chunks to take along.

But don't go overboard and take more than you
need. Remember, there are grocery stores
wherever you go, so don't bring too many perishable
foods. Call your hotel ahead of time, and request
a microwave and a refrigerator. This will minimize
your need to go out to restaurants, which is another
added stress. Some travelers opt to order

gluten-free food, and have it shipped directly to their hotel.

The following is a great list of gluten-free snacks that are perfect for travel:

Protein

- Hard-boiled eggs
- String cheese
- Beef jerky
- Hot dogs
- Canned chicken
- Tuna/salmon pouches

Fruits and Vegetables

- Pre-cut broccoli and cauliflower
- Apples
- Oranges
- Grapes
- Avocado

- Cherry tomatoes

Non-perishables

- Dried fruits
- Trail mix
- Protein bars
- Rice meals

How to Tell if a Restaurant Has Gluten-Free Options

From the outside, it can be impossible to tell if a restaurant will cater to its gluten-free patrons. But there are a few basic rules of thumb to help you along the way. Mexican, particularly authentic Mexican, usually has multiple gluten-free choices. This is because the majority uses corn to make their chips and tortillas.

Seek out local restaurants. Small, local cafes and bistros are more likely to use local ingredients, have more eclectic menus, and are more likely to offer gluten-free options. Major chains can be more difficult because their customers don't seem to have a high demand for gluten-free dishes.

However, some restaurants are noticing the growing number of gluten-free customers, and offering gluten-free options on their menu. Here is a list of popular chains that are gluten-free friendly:

- Carrabba's
- Cheeseburger in Paradise
- Chili's
- Outback Steakhouse
- On the Border
- P.F. Chang's
- Ruby Tuesday
- Uno Chicago Grill

Chapter 7:   Overcoming Obstacles

Coping Emotionally with a Gluten-Free Diet

Switching to a gluten-free diet can be very emotionally challenging during the first few weeks and months. While it can be a relief to come to your celiac or gluten-intolerant diagnosis, there is a huge shift in your everyday life.   It is not uncommon for patients to go through a grieving process as the reality of their new lifestyle sets in.   Most people experience a

combination of sadness and anger as they are adjusting. It can be frustrating and disappointing to learn that you can no longer eat some of your favorite foods.

Going to the grocery store is frequently a sensitive activity when changing to a gluten-free diet.   It can feel like torture to walk through aisles of food that you are not able to eat anymore.   Some people end up spending hours in the store, reading food labels, and still walk out unsatisfied with their purchases. Try making a list of items you know you will want before you go to the store; this will make your trip less stressful and time-consuming.

You will need to deal with your emotions regarding the foods you once loved, and can no longer eat. This proves to be particularly difficult for many people. It can be frustrating and depressing to watch your family and friends enjoy the food you want to eat, especially if you haven't found gluten-free alternatives yet. Holidays prove particularly difficult because it is possible that you are the only gluten-free eater present; and others may not know about your condition yet.

Unfortunately, the only way to deal with these situations is to remove yourself from them. Don't torture yourself by staying in the room when your friends order a pizza.   But make sure you look for other gluten-free foods that you can enjoy as well. Many restaurants now offer gluten-free pizzas.   Find out which ones in your area have gluten-free options.

Most importantly, don't take any chances if you aren't sure if a dish contains gluten.   It can be tempting, especially at first, to indulge in a treat that isn't gluten-free, but you'll regret it immensely as soon as your symptoms kick in.   And remember, ingesting gluten can do serious damage to your health.   It is easy to feel like those around you don't care about your gluten intolerance.   Rather than assuming you are being intentionally excluded, keep in mind, it's more likely that they are uneducated, not insensitive.

The first few months will undoubtedly be difficult as you transition, so expect to have some emotional swings.   Just remember it will get easier.   The longer you are on the diet the more comfortable you will become, and your mood is bound to improve.

How to Embrace the Gluten-Free Lifestyle

Going gluten-free because of dietary needs can put a real damper on food and eating.   Gluten-free diets talk a lot about what you can't have, and what gluten-free goods "aren't."   Focus instead on what they are!   There are so many different flours for gluten-free bakers to enjoy, and they each have their own distinct flavor.   On this diet, you can cater to your own specific tastes, rather than getting stuck with regular old wheat flour that is always the same. Here are a few tips to add more flavor to your gluten-free baking recipes:

- Increase the amount of extracts you use. It really adds a lot to the flavor to add some extra vanilla or almond extract.

- Use fruit and vegetable purees for some of the liquids in the recipe instead

- Use brown sugar in place of some of the granulated sugar. The molasses in the brown sugar will really punch up the flavor and moistness.

- Add more spices than the recipe calls for. If it asks for ½ tablespoon of cinnamon, double it!

Make sure you have realistic expectations when you change your diet. Some people feel better immediately after moving to a gluten-free diet. But depending on the severity of the damage done to your small intestine and how long you went undiagnosed, it may take several months to really notice the effects of a gluten-free diet.

Remember that your body still has to heal itself.

Going gluten-free can be like running a marathon. You don't get the results you want overnight! Gluten may have been just one of several allergies that your body reacted to once the damage to your intestines progressed. If symptoms are still present after a few weeks, try eliminating lactose and/or casein to see if that makes a difference. Whatever you do, don't let the sadness and frustration take over. Learn to love food again!

Chapter 8: Gluten-Free Resources
iPhone Apps

If you have ever tried shopping for gluten-free foods or wondered if a restaurant offered gluten-free menus, there's now an app for that. There are multiple apps that help you navigate what foods are gluten-free and point you in the right direction for dining out.

1. Is That Gluten Free? For Groceries. This app by Midlife Crisis Apps is designed for celiac patients, those with gluten sensitivities, and anyone interested in learning more about a gluten-free lifestyle. It includes over 14,800 verified gluten-free products from more than 360 brands. The app even includes private-label grocery store brands. Users can search ingredients to determine if a product is safe, unsafe or potentially unsafe. You can also search by category, brand or product name. The app provides links to different company websites for more

information. The cost is $7.99 with free updates and no monthly fees.

2. Is That Gluten Free? Eating Out. Also from Midlife Crisis Apps, this covers 26 national and regional restaurant chains that have gluten-free menus. The app includes fast food restaurants, like Arby's, fast casual restaurants, like Red Robin, and casual restaurants like P.F. Chang's, Red Lobster and Outback Steakhouse. The $3.99 app gives details on over 2,000 menu items at restaurants, and also offers the convenient search feature.

3. iEatOut Gluten & Allergy Free. Allergy Free Passport brings us this app that allows you to select different allergens, and provides

ingredient lists from different ethnic and international restaurant menus to decide what will be best for you.   Please note, it does not include actual restaurant menus, so talk with your waiter or the chef to ensure your meal is gluten-free.   At $4.99, the app covers Chinese, Italian, Indian, Mexican, French, Thai and Steak and Seafood restaurants.

4. Gluten-Free Groceries.   Since 2005, Triumph Dining has created print versions of their gluten-free restaurant guide and gluten-free grocery guide.   Now available in an app, it covers information on over 30,000 gluten-free products to find in the grocery store.   Users can browse by brand name, like Coca-Cola or Hidden Valley, or store

names, like Wal-Mart.   This app costs $17.99.

5. My Grocery Master.   This $1.99 app lets you search for gluten-free, kosher and lactose-free groceries.   It features more than 100,000 products from hundreds of brands.   Simply type in the desired product, category or brand name with your zip code, and the app provides you with the name of the store nearest you that carries the product you are searching for.   It also offers driving directions!   The app includes nearly all of the top 100 grocery stores in the United States, as well as Internet grocery stores.

6. Easy Gluten-Free Recipes.   Created by a working mom with three children of her own,

this app has over 100 recipes and meals that are gluten-free. It even offers specific brand names to take the hassle out of shopping and meal planning. Recipes are broken down into five categories: breakfast, lunch, dinner, snacks and desserts. Prep time for most of the meals is 15 minutes. The Easy Gluten-Free recipes app is $1.99.

7. Gluten-Free Lifestyle. Make your own grocery lists; keep track of your gluten-free food expenses for tax purposes and exchange tips and advice from others in this $1.99 app. A great feature of this app is the list of FDA recalls and food alerts.

8. Gluten-Free Restaurant Cards. This app from CeliacTravel.com is a great resource

when dining out. It includes restaurant cards in over 40 languages that you can show to your server, chef or manager to ensure you have a gluten-free meal.

Chapter 9: Celiac for College Students

The Cafeteria

Cafeteria food has a bad reputation as it is, but those with Celiac and gluten-intolerance face a unique challenge: finding foods that are safe. When choosing a college, find out everything you can about their food service program. Keep your eye open for dining services that have training programs, and ask how they accommodate students with food allergies, like yours. Be cautious of colleges with new dining managers or chefs. Chances are those who are getting a new program up and running at the beginning of the school year, special dietary needs are more likely to fall through the cracks.

Not all small colleges are a safer choice. Schools with a small gluten-free population may have minimal or no experience with serving gluten-free meals. Ask the kitchen staff specific questions about their gluten-free options, and watch for mistakes or weaknesses in their preparation processes. Some schools are very receptive and eager to help those with food allergies, and others simply are not. Before deciding on a school, try eating a meal in their dining hall, and see what options they already have available to you. You may be surprised at what you find.

Parents know your child. Is he or she comfortable asking for help with meal questions? If your child is more likely to try to ignore symptoms to blend in, look for a school that makes it easy and convenient to find gluten-free meals. Keep in mind, even freshman can be excused from living in the dorms if it is for medical reasons. Many people choose to live off-campus for this reason, as it is often the safer route. This is particularly a good choice if you, or your child, doesn't have the typical gastrointestinal symptoms, but experiences the more non-specific fatigue and flu-like symptoms.

A lot of colleges will suggest that parents take a more hands-off approach, and let their child be more independent now that they are in college. But don't let that keep you from ensuring that he or she is getting the dietary accommodations that were promised. Moreover, if your child's meal needs aren't being met, don't be afraid to ask for a refund. College meals are expensive, and you deserve to get what you paid for!

Dorm Room Survival Tips

If you have hesitations about eating in the cafeteria at school, don't give yourself anxiety by forcing yourself to eat there.   You can choose to make your own meals to eat in your dorm room or apartment.   It might not be as convenient as walking to the dining hall, but you are guaranteed you will know exactly what is in your food, and can more easily prevent cross-contamination.

When you go home for a weekend, stock up on gluten-free foods to take back with you.   Make these meals in advance and keep them in your refrigerator when you get back to school.   Take quart-size freezer bags and fill them with meals like fried rice, chicken, vegetables, and other gluten-free goodies like pizza and cookies.   Other good options to keep on hand are corn tortillas (not flour!) and shredded cheese for easily-microwavable quesadillas. Keep other foods too, that don't have to be refrigerated. Stock up on gluten-free crackers and pretzels, and other snacks like beef jerky. Specifically gluten-free foods can sometimes be more expensive, so look for foods and snacks that are already gluten free, like potato chips.

Make sure you cover your basics, like carbohydrates and protein so that you won't go hungry. The trick on a gluten-free diet is to make sure you have enough food readily available so that you don't go hungry. You should also have a variety of sauces and spices to give your food different, bolder flavors. Rice multiple times a week can get monotonous, so try new recipes to keep your food enjoyable. A few good spices and condiments to have on hand are ketchup, mustard, garlic powder, onion powder, hot sauce and mayonnaise.

Even if you do opt to eat in the cafeteria, it is still a great idea to keep several gluten-free food options in your room. Late-night study sessions are inevitable—and so is the need for some late night snacks. Taking a risk with gluten foods isn't worth it to satisfy a craving. Always stock up!

Social Struggles

Starting college means meeting new people, a lot of new people, for the first time. Whether you want to draw attention to your celiac or gluten-intolerance or not, people are bound to notice you eating your cheeseburger without the bun. For some people it can be embarrassing, or simply frustrating, to have to explain your allergy to people so often. Look at it as an opportunity to educate others on celiac and the effects of gluten.

Learning to socialize with celiac can be complicated as well. It's not a secret that college is a time when people party. And on a college budget, a party means beer. For celiac patients and others with a gluten sensitivity or gluten intolerance, beer is out of the question. It can make you feel like a dud to have to turn down beer after beer, or annoyed explaining your allergy every time. But there are plenty of alternatives to beer. Don't hesitate to bring your own beverages, like hard ciders or gluten-free liquors.

Most people don't expect how many events and functions are planned around food in college. From hanging out with friends to important meetings, banquets and dinners, most of these involve food. You may try suffering through boring salads and water the first few times, but that is bound to get old.   Ask a server or the dining staff if they have any grilled vegetables or chicken in the kitchen that they could offer you.   Don't let yourself feel like a burden for asking for these alternatives; if anything, your celiac or gluten-intolerance is a burden that you can't control. Remember, you have the right to eat what your body needs.

Chapter 10:   Quick Facts on Celiac and Gluten Sensitivity/Intolerance

- Celiac is an autoimmune disorder that damages the small intestine and interferes with your body's ability to absorb the nutrients from food.

- 30-40% of Americans have a genetic predisposition to develop celiac.   This is the equivalent of 1 in every 133 people.

- Only 1% will actually develop the disease.

- Roughly 95% of celiac patients are undiagnosed or misdiagnosed.

- On average, it takes 6-10 years for a person to be correctly diagnosed with celiac.

- 5-22% of people with celiac have another immediate family member who also has the disease.

- There are over 300 symptoms tied to celiac and gluten sensitivity and gluten intolerance.

- There is a 1 in 39 chance that people who have second-degree relatives with the disease will have celiac.

- 1 in 236 people of African American, Hispanic or Asian American descent will have celiac.

- Celiac can lead to infertility, reduced bone density, some cancers, neurological disorders, and other autoimmune diseases.

- 610,000 women in America experience unexplained infertility; 6% (36,600) will never learn that celiac is the cause.

- There is no pharmaceutical cure for celiac.

- The only treatment for celiac disease is a strict, entirely gluten-free diet.

- Due to raising public awareness, it is estimated that by 2019, 50-60% of the population will be diagnosed with celiac.

- Gluten-free food sales reached $2.6 billion in 2010, and are believed to exceed $5 billion by 2015.

- In the United States, 3 million people have Type 1 Diabetes, and 6% (180,000) of them also have celiac.

- 12% (42,000) of the 350,000 people in America living with Down syndrome also have celiac.

- Celiac disease occurs in 20% of people who have collagenous colitis
- Children born to women who have celiac or other gluten sensitivities may be at a higher risk for developing schizophrenia and other psychiatric diseases later in life.
- 60% of children and 41% of adults do not show symptoms of celiac.
- Only 35% of newly diagnosed patients list chronic diarrhea as a symptom, doing away with the theory that diarrhea must be present to diagnose celiac.
- Children diagnosed with celiac between ages 2 and 4 have a 10.5% chance of developing another autoimmune disorder; 16.7% chance between 4-12; 27% chance from ages 12-20, and a 34% chance over 20 years of age.

- The number of people with celiac in America is almost equal to the population of the state of Nevada.

Chapter 11:   Gluten-Free Recipes

Gluten-Free Chocolate Chip Cookies

Ingredients:

- 8 ounces unsalted butter
- 2 cups (11 ounces) brown white flour
- ¼ cup (1 ¼ ounces) cornstarch
- 2 tbsp. (½ ounce) tapioca flour
- 1 tsp. xanthan gum
- 1 tsp. kosher salt
- 1 tsp. baking soda
- ¼ cup (2 ounces) sugar
- 1 ¼ cup (10 ounces) light brown sugar
- 1 whole egg
- 1 egg yolk
- 2 tbsp whole milk
- 1 ½ teaspoons vanilla extract

- 12 ounces semisweet chocolate chips

Directions:

Preheat your oven to 375 degrees F.

Over low heat, melt the butter in a heavy-bottom medium saucepan.   Once this is melted, pour it into a stand mixer bowl.

Sift together the rice flour, cornstarch, tapioca flour, xanthan, salt and baking soda in a medium bowl. Set these ingredients aside.

Add the sugar and brown sugar to the bowl with butter.   Use the paddle attachment to mix the ingredients together on medium speed for one minute.   Add the egg yolk, milk and vanilla extract, and mix until they are combined.   Finally, add the chocolate chips.

Let the dough chill in the refrigerator for approximately one hour, or until the dough is firm. Form the dough into 2-ounce balls and place on a cookie sheet lined with parchment paper. Bake for 14 minutes, rotating halfway through for even baking. Remove cookies from the oven and let cool for two minutes. Then, move the cookies to a wire cooling rack to cool completely. Store the cookies in an airtight container.

Nutritional Information (per cookie):

- Calories: 251
- Total fat: 13 grams
- Saturated fat: 7.5 grams
- Protein: 2 grams
- Total Carbohydrates: 35 grams
- Sugar: 22 grams
- Fiber: 2 grams

- Cholesterol: 38 milligrams
- Sodium: 143 milligrams

Garden Vegetable Soup

Ingredients:

- 4 tbsp. olive oil
- 2 cups chopped leeks (white part only)
- 2 tbsp. finely minced garlic
- Kosher salt
- 2 cups carrots, peeled and chopped into rounds
- 2 cups peeled and diced potatoes
- 2 cups fresh green beans, broken or cut into ¾-inch pieces
- 2 quarts chicken or vegetable broth
- 4 cups peeled, seeded and chopped tomatoes
- 2 ears of corn, kernels removed
- ½ tsp. freshly ground black pepper
- ¼ cup packed, chopped fresh parsley leaves

- 1-2 tsp. freshly squeezed lemon juice

Directions:

Heat the olive oil in a large, heavy bottom stockpot over medium-low heat. Once the oil is hot, add the leeks, garlic and a pinch of salt until they begin to soften. This should take approximately 7-8 minutes. Next, add the carrots, potatoes and green beans and continue cooking 4-5 minutes, stirring occasionally.

Add the chicken or vegetable stock, increase the heat, and bring to a simmer. Then add the tomatoes, corn kernels and pepper. Reduce the heat to low, cover, and cook 25-30 minutes, or until the vegetables are tender enough to be cut with a fork. Remove from the heat, and add the lemon juice and parsley. Add salt to taste. Serve immediately. Makes six servings.

Nutritional Information:

- Calories: 255
- Total fat: 12 grams
- Saturated fat: 1 gram
- Protein: 6 grams
- Total carbohydrates: 33 grams
- Sugar: 8 grams
- Fiber: 6 grams
- Cholesterol: 0 milligrams
- Sodium: 1385 milligrams

Recipe copyright: Food Network

Slow-Cooker Pork Tacos

Ingredients:

- 3 whole ancho chilies

- 3 whole pasilla chilies
- 4 cloves garlic, unpeeled
- 2-3 chipotles in adobo sauce
- ½ medium white onion, roughly chopped
- 3 tbsp. extra-virgin olive oil
- 2 tbsp. honey
- 1 tbsp. cider vinegar
- Kosher salt
- 2 tsp. dried oregano, preferably Mexican oregano
- 3 ¾ cups low-sodium chicken broth
- 4 lbs. boneless pork shoulder (untrimmed), cut into chunks
- Freshly ground pepper
- 2 bay leaves
- 1 cinnamon stick
- Corn tortillas, warmed for serving
- Assorted taco toppings

Directions:

In a microwave-safe bowl, microwave the ancho and pasilla chilies and garlic on high for 2-3 minutes, or until soft and pliable.   Stem and seed the chilies, and peel the garlic.   Transfer the chilies and garlic into a blender.

Add the chipotles, onion, 2 tbsp. of olive oil, honey, vinegar, 1 tbsp. salt and the oregano to the blender and puree until smooth.   Heat the remaining 1 tbsp. of oil in a large skillet over high heat.   Add the chili sauce and fry, stirring for about 8 minutes, or until thick and fragrant.   Add the broth and reduce the heat until it is slightly thickened.

Season the pork shoulder with salt and pepper, and transfer to a slow cooker.   Add the bay leaves and cinnamon stick, and then pour the sauce over top. Cover and cook on high for approximately 5 hours,

or until the meat is tender. If you don't have a
slow cooker, you can cook the meat in a Dutch oven,
covered, for 1 hour and 45 minutes at 350 degrees.
Then, uncover and cook an additional 30 minutes.

Once the meat is cooked, discard the cinnamon and
bay leaves. Shred the pork with two forks and
season with salt and pepper. Serve the shredded
pork in the warmed corn tortillas along with your
additional toppings. Serves 8.

Nutritional Information (does not include tortillas
or garnishes):

- Calories: 399
- Total fat: 15 grams
- Saturated fat: 4 grams
- Protein: 51 grams
- Total carbohydrates: 14 grams
- Sugar: 5 grams

- Fiber: 3 grams

- Cholesterol: 147 milligrams

- Sodium: 212 milligrams

Grilled Sweet Potatoes with Lime and Cilantro

Ingredients:

- 3 sweet potatoes, unpeeled
- Kosher salt
- 2 tsp. finely grated lime zest
- Pinch cayenne pepper
- ¼ cup canola oil
- Freshly ground pepper
- ¼ cup finely chopped fresh cilantro

Directions:

Place the sweet potatoes in a pot of water and boil until they are fork-tender; let cool. Slice each sweet potato lengthwise into 8 pieces.

Preheat your grill to medium heat or use a cast-iron grill pan over a medium heat stove. Mix the lime zest, 1 tbsp. salt and cayenne in a small bowl. Brush the potato wedges with the oil and season with salt and pepper. Grill until cooked all the way through and are golden brown and both sides. Transfer to a platter and immediately season with the salt mixture. Sprinkle with cilantro. Serves 4.

Nutritional Information:

- Calories: 209
- Total fat: 14 grams
- Saturated fat: 1 gram
- Protein: 2 grams
- Total carbohydrates: 20 grams

- Sugar: 4 grams

- Fiber: 3 grams

- Cholesterol: 0 milligrams

- Sodium: 174 milligrams

Hummus Dip

Ingredients:

- 2 (15 ounce) cans chickpeas, rinsed and drained

- ½ cup extra virgin olive oil, or more as needed

- ½ lemon, juiced

- 2 tbsp. roughly chopped fresh parsley leaves

- 2 cloves garlic, peeled

- 1 ½ tsp. salt

- ½ tsp. dark Asian sesame oil

- ½-1 tsp. ground cumin

- 12-15 grinds black pepper

- ¼ cup water

- Paprika, for garnish

Directions:

Combine all ingredients in a blender except for the parsley and paprika.   Blend together on a slow speed until smooth.   You will have to stop the blender frequently to scrape the ingredients off the side.   If the mixture is too dry to blend, add a few more tablespoons of olive oil.

Scrape the hummus onto a plate.   Sprinkle the paprika over the top and drizzle with more olive oil. Place parsley on top for garnish.   If you make the dip ahead, cover with plastic wrap and leave at room temperature.

Nutritional Information (per tablespoon):

- Calories: 57

- Total fat: 4 grams

- Saturated fat: .5 grams

- Protein: 1 gram

- Total carbohydrates: 5 grams

- Sugar: 0 grams

- Fiber: 1 gram

- Cholesterol: 0 milligrams

- Sodium: 96 milligrams

Recipe copyright: Food Network

Quinoa Tabbouleh

Ingredients:

- ½ cup quinoa (red or white), rinsed

- ½ cup freshly squeezed lemon juice

- ¼ cup extra virgin olive oil

- Kosher salt

- Freshly ground pepper

- Pinch of freshly grated nutmeg

- 3 bunches fresh, flat-leaf parsley, finely chopped (about 4 cups), best results when cut by hand
- ½ cup finely chopped fresh mint leaves
- 1 pint cherry tomatoes, quartered
- 1 English cucumber, diced
- Small handful jarred peppadew peppers and roasted red peppers, finely chopped

Directions:

Bring one cup of water to boil in a small saucepan. At the same time, toast the quinoa in a small cast-iron skillet over medium-high heat. The grains will give off a nutty scent and begin to pop. Pour the quinoa into the boiling water. Turn the water down to a simmer, cover and cook until the water is absorbed and the quinoa is tender. This should take 12-15 minutes. Remove from heat and allow it to cool.

Whisk the olive oil, lemon juice, ½ rounded teaspoon of salt, pepper and nutmeg together. In a large bowl, combine the parsley, mint, cherry tomatoes, cucumber, peppadews, and cooled cooked quinoa. Pour the dressing over the salad and toss to coat thoroughly. Taste for seasoning and let sit for five minutes before you serve. Serves 6.

Nutritional Information

- Calories: 175
- Total Fat: 10 grams
- Saturated fat: 1.5 grams
- Protein: 4 grams
- Total carbohydrates: 17 grams
- Sugar: 4 grams
- Fiber: 3.5 grams
- Cholesterol: 0 milligrams
- Sodium: 170 milligrams

Berry Pavlovas

Ingredients:

- ½ cup sugar
- 2 egg whites
- 1 tsp. cornstarch
- ½ tsp. vanilla extract
- ½ tsp. distilled white vinegar
- ½ cup heavy cream
- 1 cup sliced strawberries
- ¼ cup apricot jam
- 2 tbsp. hot water

Directions:

Preheat your oven to 275 degrees F. Cover a large baking sheet with parchment paper.

Pulse the sugar in a food processor to make it fine, or just buy extra-fine sugar, and set it aside. In a medium glass bowl, whip the eggs on a low speed until they are foamy. Add half of the sugar and continue to whip until stiff peaks form. In a small bowl, sift the remaining sugar with the cornstarch. Add this to the egg whites, as well as the vanilla and vinegar. Blend until incorporated.

Spoon the mixture into 4 piles on the covered baking sheet. Use a spoon to create a hollowed out section in pile. Bake for 40 minutes; turn off the oven and let the pavlovas in the oven untouched for another 20 minutes. Remove from the oven and allow cooling.

Whip the cream until it makes soft peaks. Top the cooled pavlovas with whipped cream and strawberries.

Make a quick sauce by thinning the apricot jam with the hot water, and drizzle over the pavlovas.   Serves 4.

Nutritional Information:

- Calories: 274
- Total fat: 11 grams
- Saturated fat: 7 grams
- Protein: 3 grams
- Total carbohydrates: 43 grams
- Sugar: 36 grams
- Fiber: 1 gram
- Cholesterol: 41 milligrams
- Sodium: 48 milligrams

Frittata with Asparagus, Tomato and Fontina

Ingredients:

- 6 large eggs

- 2 tbsp. whipping cream
- ½ tsp. salt, plus a pinch
- ¼ tsp. freshly ground black pepper
- 1 tbsp. olive oil
- 1 tbsp. butter
- 12 oz. asparagus, trimmed, cut into ¼-½ inch pieces
- 1 tomato, seeded and diced
- Salt
- 3 oz. Fontina, diced

Directions:

Preheat the broiler.   In a medium bowl, whisk the eggs, cream, ½ tsp. of salt and pepper, and set aside. Heat the oil and butter in a 9 ½ inch, non-stick ovenproof skillet over medium heat.   Next, add the asparagus and sauté for approximately 2 minutes, or until crisp and tender.   Raise the heat to medium-high, and add the tomato and a pinch of salt; sauté two minutes longer.

Pour the egg mixture over the asparagus mixture and cook until the eggs begin to set.   Sprinkle over top with cheese.   Reduce the heat to medium-low and continue cooking until the frittata is almost set, but the top is still runny.   Place the skillet under the broil, and broil until the top is set and golden brown; this should take about five minutes.   Let the frittata stand 2 minutes.   Loosen the frittata from the skillet with a rubber spatula and slide onto a plate.   Serves 6.

Nutritional Information:

- Calories: 197
- Total fat: 15 grams
- Saturated fat: 7 grams
- Protein: 11 grams
- Total carbohydrates: 4 grams

- Sugar: 2 grams

- Fiber: 1 gram

- Cholesterol: 214 milligrams

- Sodium: 351 milligrams

Recipe copyright: Food Network

Spring Garden Potato Salad

Ingredients:

Dressing:

- 2 cloves garlic, peeled

- 2 ½ tsp. kosher salt

- ½ cup mayonnaise

- 2 ½ tbsp. white wine vinegar

- Freshly ground black pepper

Salad:

- 8 cups water

- 2/3 cup dry white vermouth

- 3 cloves garlic, smashed
- 2 tbsp. kosher salt, plus additional for seasoning
- 1 sprig fresh thyme
- 1 bay leaf
- 4 black peppercorns
- 2 lbs. small red-skinned, waxy potatoes, sliced into 1/8 inch thick rounds
- 5 medium carrots, peeled and sliced into 1/8 inch thick rounds
- 1 bunch radishes, sliced into 1/8 inch thick rounds (about 8 radishes)
- ½ English cucumber or 1 large Kirby cucumber, sliced into 1/8 inch thick rounds
- 1 cup grape or cherry tomatoes, halved
- 3 scallions (white and green parts), thinly sliced
- Freshly ground black pepper
- ½ cup lightly packed mixed fresh herbs, such as flat leaf parsley, dill or tarragon
- 6 lemon wedges

Directions:

Dressing—smash the garlic cloves and then sprinkle the salt overtop. Work the mixture until you have a coarse paste. Add this to the mayonnaise, vinegar and black pepper in a small bowl and whisk it together.

Salad in a large saucepan, bring the water, vermouth, garlic, salt, thyme, bay leaf, peppercorns and potatoes to a boil. Add the carrots, lower the heat, and cook for about five minutes, or until the vegetables are tender. Stir in the radishes, and then drain all the vegetables right away. Remove and throw away the garlic, thyme, bay leaf and peppercorns. Allow to cool briefly and then toss the vegetables with the dressing. Cover and refrigerate for about a half hour.

About 10 minutes before serving, combine the cucumber, tomatoes, and scallions in a bowl with salt and pepper to your preference.   When you are ready to serve the salad, add the cucumber mixture and herbs into the potato salad and serve with lemon wedges.   Serves 6.

Nutritional Information:

- Calories: 280
- Total fat: 15 grams
- Saturated fat: 2 grams
- Protein: 4 grams
- Total carbohydrates: 33 grams
- Sugar: 6 grams
- Fiber: 5 grams
- Cholesterol: 7 milligrams
- Sodium: 2,910 milligrams

Chapter 12:   Testimonial

Lizzy Sulkowski

Lizzy Sulkowski was diagnosed with gluten intolerance when she was 23.   When she first noticed the symptoms, she was unsure what could be wrong with her.   Within three months she had lost twenty pounds, and was experiencing major stomach discomfort on an almost daily basis. Initially, she tried to self-diagnose what could be wrong, believing it was first alcohol intolerance, and then lactose intolerance.   When cutting alcohol and dairy from her diet didn't change or even slow her symptoms, she cut out gluten to see if it would make a difference.   As it seemed to help, she visited a gastroenterologist to confirm what she believed was causing her to experience the symptoms she had.

After an extensive diagnostic process, including a biopsy and endoscopy, she was diagnosed as gluten intolerant.   This is her account of how switching to a gluten-free diet has affected her life:

Switching to gluten free actually taught me to more easily balance my emotions. Physically, I felt better; but emotionally, I was struggling. Some people don't believe in a gluten intolerance or a gluten allergy. It was a difficult transition in my social life. I had to change all of the drinks I was drinking, (including alcohol) and all of the food I ordered when I went out to eat. Ordering food was intense for me. I felt like I was putting people out or causing them more struggle by ordering gluten-free. I had to learn how to settle into my food intolerance. I'm doing much better with it now. It helps to live in an area with local restaurants that tend to cater to the local people, rather than the overall demographic.

It also took a toll on me because I was changing on the outside. I lost more weight, and the more weight I lost...

well. More people noticed. I had a hard time explaining what my very new body was going through. I have finally found a "synergy" between my emotions, body, and food. Having the gluten allergy forces you to take a healthier route with food.

The changes I've noticed are mostly in my physical body and overall attentiveness. I'm less tired and more energized. I eat more frequently than I use to. It's also easier to make room for food that doesn't make you extremely full. You get to enjoy and eat a little bit more than the average gluten-consumer.

Some of the most difficult aspects of eating food without gluten was finding food that still made me feel full and energized. If you're an active person with a gluten allergy, you have to almost eat twice as much as the next person. Another difficult thing to adjust to was eating out. Having a gluten allergy means that you have to learn how to cook for yourself. A lot of restaurants still don't cater to a gluten allergy. My advice? Find ones that do. It's more common to find gluten free-foods at local restaurants.

I learned to cope with finding treats that are some of my vices. One of my vices is chocolate. Most chocolate is gluten-free. I also learned the beauty of the rice crispy treat - very easy to make and pretty cheap for purchase. You can pile on pretty much anything to a rice crispy. I also found a love for sugared fruits. Any frozen fruit is fantastic.

Embracing a gluten-free diet is just that. Embracing it. Embrace yourself. Remind yourself that a gluten allergy is not your "fault." It's just a little different from the rest of the world. Search for foods that make you happy. Search for

foods that fill you up.